DRJOH

You Don't Need Your Glasses or Contacts

Natural Ways to Correct Your Vision Without Drugs or Corrective Lenses

Dr John DeWitt

Corrective lenses are a crutch that we don't have to depend on. These simple exercises can allow you to see better and eliminate the need for glasses or contacts. I have personally seen the benefits and encourage my patients to use them.

drjohndewitt.com

You Don't Need Your Glasses or Contacts

drjohndewitt.com

drjohndewitt.com

Contents

Disclaimer 11
IMPROVE YOUR EYESIGHT NATURALLY WITH THE BATES METHOD 12
Glasses Since 8th Grade 22
The Crux of Bates teachings 25
    Who is this book for? 26
    What you can potentially gain from the exercises? 27
    How to Begin 27
    How long is a daily practice? 31
    What if my eyes feel fatigued? 31
    How long before I see improved vision? ... 32
    Do I just stop wearing my glasses? 32
    How long does it take before one can throw away their glasses? 32
    What kinds of eye problems can be corrected with the Bates Method? 33
    Is recovery of good vision possible? 34
    Does my vision remain constant? 34
    What Bates Methods will I learn? 34
Eye Anatomy 37
How Vision Works 38
BATES EXERCISES 42
    Relaxation 42

Signs that your eyes are strained. 42
Breathing 44
    Exercise One: Deep Breathing 45
    Exercise Two: Lens Flexor.................... 46
Stretching 48
Movement.. 50
    Exercise One: Sway 51
    Exercise Two: Long Swing 53
        Benefits of the long swing...................... 54
        Exercise One 59
        Exercise Two 62
        Exercise Three 64
        Exercise Four 67
Energetic Yawning.................................... 70
Blinking.. 71
Palming 74
    How to Palm 76
When to Palm 82
How long to Palm 83
What to do if you can't relax 85
Sunning... 86
    Sunning benefits:.................................. 90
How to do basic sunning 91
Advanced sunning techniques 95

drjohndewitt.com

You Don't Need Your Glasses or Contacts

How long to sun for 96
When to sun... 97
What to do after sunning 98
    Blink:... 98
    Palm:... 99
Pinhole Glasses...................................... 103
Alternate Eye Movements......................... 106
Lazy Eights 110
Central Fixation... 113
    Exercise One: Tibetan Wheel 116
    Exercise 2: Snellen Chart 118
    Exercise Three: Domino Chart............... 120
    Exercise Four: Edging 122
    Exercise Five: Mandala 126
Fusion 128
    Exercise 1 131
    Exercise 2:..133
    Exercise 3...134
Eye Oblique Muscle Stretch 136
Near / Far Exercise 138
Eye-Mind Connection 140
Visualization...142
    Exercise 1: Ship sailing out....................142
    Exercise 2: Runners on the track...........145

drjohndewitt.com

Analytic Vision 148
Nutrition 152
    Vitamin A 152
    Vitamin C 153
    Vitamin E: 153
    Antioxidants: 154
    DHA, Omega-3s: 154
    Zinc: 155
20 Surprising Foods to Promote Eye Health 156
    Leafy Greens 158
    Eggs 158
    Citrus fruits 160
    Seeds and nuts 160
    Wild Blueberries 161
    Sweet Potatoes 163
    Fatty Fish 163
    Whole Grains 164
    Legumes 165
    Grass Fed Beef 166
    Coconut Milk 167
    Tomatoes 168
    Olive Oil 169
    Non-GMO Corn 170

Pistachios 171
Strawberries 172
Avocado 173
Peppers 173
Dark Chocolate 174
Tea and Coffee 175
Chiropractic Care and your Vision – What's the Connection? 178
SUMMING UP 187
Bates Exercises...Overview 188
   Relaxation 188
      Breathing: 188
      Stretching: 188
Movement: 189
   Energetic Yawning: 189
   Blinking: 189
   Palming: 190
   Sunning: 190
   Pinhole Glasses: 191
   Alternate Eye Movements: 191
   Lazy Eights 191
   Central Fixation 192
   Fusion 193
   Eye Oblique Muscle Stretch 194

drjohndewitt.com

    Near / Far 194
    Eye-Mind Connection 194
    Analytic Vision 195
    Nutrition 196
    Foods for Better Vision 196
    Chiropractic 198
Conclusion 198
DAILY PRACTICE 199
Resources 201

Disclaimer

I am not certified as a Bates practitioner, a Medical Doctor or Optometrist. I believe in natural ways to heal the body by working with the body's ability to heal itself. I am a Chiropractor that has experienced the results of these exercises and only wish to share this information with others so that they may benefit from them as well.

IMPROVE YOUR EYESIGHT NATURALLY WITH THE BATES METHOD

Wouldn't it be great to see clearly without glasses or contacts? The good news is almost everyone can, even those of you already wearing strong corrective lenses. The secret lies in a method developed in the 19th century.

Over 100 years ago, Dr. William H Bates began investigating the causes of poor sight. He came up with a radical (to traditionalists) method to improve vision for short sight, long sight, astigmatism, 'old-age sight', squint, 'lazy' eye, and even structural diseases such as macular degeneration. What was the essence of his work? Learning to use the eyes normally and, more importantly to relax them. It was as simple as that. To do this, he devised different exercises and found them to improve different vision problems to where his patients no longer needed to rely on wearing glasses.

A fully trained ophthalmologist, in the late 1800s he ran his practice conventionally. He put people in glasses and told them nothing different could be done. Then, for an unknown reason, he radically changed his opinion to the opposite view.

Not surprisingly, his radical new view was rejected. It was not that he didn't have good credentials and an audience. He had discovered the properties of adrenalin, and, as a surgeon, he pioneered an ear operation for deafness still used today. In truth, his colleagues thought him a brilliant man, a revolutionary who was pushing the edge of knowledge. Still, his view about correcting vision went to beyond the conventional wisdom for acceptance and there were on-going efforts to discredit him. He stayed resolute until his death in 1931. Today, the people who stand on Bates' shoulders are rarely medical people but educators.

After Bates' death, several court cases ensued to try and discredit his Method. One prominent one was with Margaret

Corbett, one of his students who was taken to court on two occasions in the 1940s charged with practicing medicine without a license. One charge brought against her claimed that she advocated a practice that would lead to retinal burns. Three hundred witnesses appeared in her defense, some Hollywood stars. All were tested and found to have healthy retinas. Able to successfully prove that what she had been doing was educating people about their eyes, she was acquitted on both occasions.

Nevertheless, such opposition by the powers that be took its toll. Bates practitioners were advised not to advertise. Even today, they practice with caution. Though thousands of anecdotal testimonials exist of the validity of the method for improving vision to where one does not need to wear glasses, including myself (more on that in a minute) little research was done to test the method and Bates Method was largely ignored.

Then in 1978, PhD student M.H. McClay conducted a two year study at the Vision Training Institute for his dissertation. He found all subjects improved significantly in their visual acuity (sharpness of vision), both nearsighted and far sighted subjects. Three people in the study, ages 51, 57, and 66 achieved normal vision, something thought not possible as the aging eye was assumed to lose near vision (presbyopia). This would not have surprised Bates, who said presbyopia is not caused by old age but by **tension**.

Other studies have been done since then but none have scientifically established improved eyesight. Several of Bates' techniques, including "sunning", "swinging", and "palming", were combined with healthy changes to diet and exercise in a 1983 study of myopic children in India. After 6 months, the experimental groups did not show any statistically significant difference in refractive status. The children in the treatment group however described relief of eye strain and other symptoms.

In 2004, the American Academy of Ophthalmology (AAO) published a review of various research on visual training, consisting of "eye exercises, muscle relaxation techniques, biofeedback, eye patches, or eye massages, alone or in combinations." None of the studies found evidence that such techniques could benefit eyesight. Some however noted changes, positive and negative, in the visual acuity of nearsighted subjects. In some cases, improvements remained at subsequent follow-ups. These results though were not viewed as actual reversals of nearsightedness, but to factors such as "improvements in interpreting blurred images, changes in mood or motivation, creation of an artificial contact lens by tear film changes, or a pinhole effect from miosis of the pupil."

In 2005 the Ophthalmology Department of New Zealand's Christchurch Hospital published a review of forty-three studies on the use of eye exercises. They found no clear scientific evidence supporting the use of eye exercises to improve visual acuity, and concluded that "their use therefore remains controversial."

These results discount all the many testimonials of the Bates Method success, perhaps the most notable being that of British writer Aldous Huxley, author of *Brave New World.* As a result of keratitis at age sixteen, Huxley suffered an 18-month period of near-blindness that left him with one eye just capable of light perception and the other with poor vision from hyperopia and astigmatism. Only by wearing thick glasses and dilating his better pupil with atropine was he able to read. At age 45, Margaret Corbett gave him regular lessons in the Bates Method. It was so successful that later he wrote *The Art of Seeing*. In this book, he relates his experiences: "Within a couple of months I was reading without spectacles and, what was better still, **without strain and fatigue**.... At the present time, my vision, though very far from normal, is about twice as good as it used to be when I wore spectacles." He concluded that: "Vision is not won by making an effort to get it: it comes to those who have learned to put their minds and eyes into a state of alert passivity, of dynamic relaxation."

Glasses Since 8th Grade

I always thought the kids that wore glasses looked smart. I remember sitting in the cafeteria in the first grade and wishing I wore glasses. I also thought the same about braces but thankfully, my parents thought better of it! I didn't actually "need" glasses until I was in the 8th grade. The frames I picked are comical as I look back today.

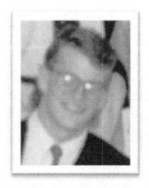

I didn't mind the glasses until I started having problems seeing while I was playing football. I played for Vanderbilt University and then 12 years of professional football after that. I needed every advantage out on the field so I wore contact lenses. This was a huge annoyance as I seemed to constantly get poked in the eye. If only I had known then what I know now!

I learned about the Bates Method about two years ago and decided to try it out immediately. Now I may be a special case…but after doing some of the exercises in this book ONCE, I was able to see clearly without glasses for the next two years!

The effects did start to wear off as time went by and I have had to revisit the exercises to get my vision "back in check". The reason I wrote this book is because I have first-hand experience with the great results that are possible and I had to share that with those of you that suffer with glasses and contacts every day just like I did.

Once again, I need to stress that I believe in natural ways to heal the body by working with the body's ability to heal itself. I am a Chiropractor that has experienced the results of these exercises and only wish to share this information with others so that they may benefit from them as well.

The Crux of Bates teachings

- Weak muscles are not the cause of poor vision. **Tense eyes are the cause** so you have to relax your eyes. The Bates Method teaches you to relax the muscles around your eyes to allow your eyes to move and function optimally.
- Stress squeezes muscles around your eyeballs and contorts them. Such strain reduces your visual acuity by altering where the field of vision lands on your retina.
- Far-sightedness, near-sightedness, astigmatism, cross-eye, glaucoma, cataracts, and other conditions can benefit from the Bates Method.

Who is this book for?

- Anyone from 5 to 100 who wishes to make their vision better as it's never too late to do so.
- Anyone who has problems with seeing correctly and wants to be able to do so.
- Anyone who uses weak, moderate or even strong reading glasses, or even bifocals or trifocals.
- Anyone who experiences eye strain, fatigue, or headaches when reading or trying to focus on the computer screen.
- Anyone with excellent near-point vision who wishes to keep it that way and save themselves from having to

wear glasses.

What you can potentially gain from the exercises?

- Freedom from reading glasses.
- A weaker prescription and more independence from reading aids.
- An improvement in any other visual condition.
- Clearer night vision.
- Less stress and more relaxation.

How to Begin

- Read the first this book
- Find out from your doctor what your special vision problem is if you a have one.

drjohndewitt.com

- Do the relaxation exercises before the eye exercises.
- Do not wear your glasses during the exercises unless your doctor advises you to do so. If so, find out which are the appropriate eyeglasses to wear.
- Make sure you have the appropriate light during your transition from wearing glasses, and especially while reading.

HELPFUL HINT: *Take frequent vision breaks throughout the day, especially during computer work or if you begin to feel any eyestrain and do the following:*

- Take off your glasses.
- Yawn three times or more (more on this later)
- Stretch your body up.
- Stretch your eye muscles by looking up, down, left, right, diagonally and around in circles.
- Shift focus quickly from near to distant objects 5 times (called shifting)
- Blink for 15 seconds or longer (tears create a natural contact lens)

- Palm for 5 deep breaths (details to come)

At first, it will be an effort to do the exercises without your glasses. But after a week or so, your eyes will be invigorated and you will see more clearly what was blurry or even invisible before.

How long is a daily practice?

That's up to you. You should practice for at least five minutes a day, ideally 15 minutes a day or longer. Obviously, the longer you devote to the exercises, the quicker you will see results.

That said, you should start out slowly and work up to a longer time. The number one rule is to **relax**, not strain your eyes! Understanding this and doing it is your key to success.

What if my eyes feel fatigued?

If you feel fatigued from the exercises, stop them for a week or so and start again. If your eyes still feel fatigued, stop them for a few weeks and begin again.

How long before I see improved vision?

In general, after around two weeks or so, you should begin to see signs of improved vision. I was lucky enough to see great results after only one session!

Do I just stop wearing my glasses?

If you have a mild prescription, gradually go more and more frequently without glasses as you feel your eyesight improving. Always, of course, wear glasses for driving if they were needed to pass your driver's test.

How long does it take before one can throw away their glasses?

The Bates Method may take some time

and you will need patience. How long varies greatly from person to person. I may have been a special case. Typically, you will need to continue the program for weeks or months, or even longer for extreme conditions.

What kinds of eye problems can be corrected with the Bates Method?

The Bates Method is successful for correcting the two most common eyesight conditions requiring glasses: myopia (near-sightedness) that typically appears in childhood or adolescence; and presbyopia (farsightedness that leads to reading glasses at middle age).

Is recovery of good vision possible?

Just as a broken limb can be rehabilitated through exercise, Bates believed that the eyes can as well. He felt that wearing glasses was the same thing as using a crutch for a broken leg.

Does my vision remain constant?

How clearly you see varies according to your physical and emotional state. In other words, vision is constantly varying.

What Bates Methods will I learn?

- Relaxation of body and eyes
    - Breathing

- Exercise One: Deep Breathing
- Exercise Two: Lens Flexor
  - Stretching
  - Body Movement
    - Exercise One: Sway
    - Exercise Two: Long Swing
    - Exercise Three: Cross-Crawl
  - Energetic Yawning
  - Blinking
  - Palming
  - Sunning (my favorite!)
  - Pinhole glasses
  - Alternate Eye Movements
- Lazy Eights

- Central fixation
    - Exercise 1: Tibetan Wheel
    - Exercise 2: Snellen Chart
    - Exercise 3: Domino Chart
    - Exercise 4: Edging
    - Exercise 5: Mandala
- Eye Oblique Stretch
- Near & Far
- Visualization
- Analytic seeing

Eye Anatomy

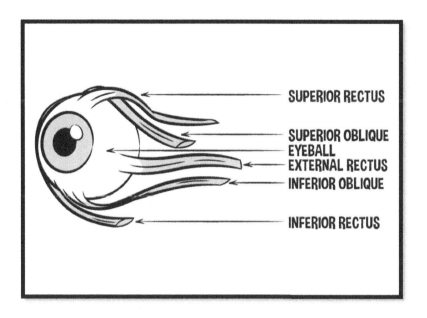

There are 6 extraocular muscles that control eye movement. These are the muscles that the Bates Method focuses on to ensure relaxed, clear vision. The image above does not show the internal (medial) rectus muscle, which pulls the eye toward the nose.

drjohndewitt.com

How Vision Works

The most common vision problems are near sightedness (can only see close objects) and farsightedness (can only see far objects). These are caused by a shift in the focal point inside the eye itself. These conditions are all based by a "short" or "long" eyeball due to muscle imbalances.

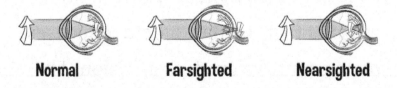

Normal   **Farsighted**   **Nearsighted**

Notice how, in normal vision, the image is focused on the retina as it should be. In farsighted people, the image has a focal point behind the retina and, in nearsighted people, it is in front of the retina.

The Visual Center is the area in the brain where images are processed. Certain chiropractic techniques can increase circulation to that area thus improving its function. See the illustration on the next page.

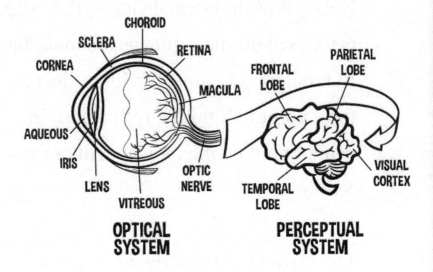

VISUAL SYSTEM

Notes

BATES EXERCISES

Relaxation

Everything about the Bates Method is about relaxing the eyes and for good reason. Normal eyes are relaxed eyes. Visions should feel effortless. Strain, whether physical, mental, emotional or spiritual will impair proper vision.

Signs that your eyes are strained.

- Squinting eyes
- Ruffled brow (causes wrinkles too!)
- Tense facial muscles
- Clenched jaw
- Mental stress

WATCH OUT: *When people have a hard time seeing they typically will squint, which actually makes your vision worse. Squinting is one of the worst things you can do for your vision as it stresses your muscles.*

If you are like the average, stressed out person living in our hectic world, good chance that you experience one or more of these signs of eye strain. You don't have to. In this guide, you will learn how to use the Bates Method to relax your eyes. In so doing, your mind and body will relax as all work together: when relaxed, your muscles lose their tension, your breath slows down and deepens, your heart rate lowers, and your vision becomes clearer and sharper.

Breathing

For the eyes to function normally, sufficient oxygen must get to them. This can only be done through deep breathing as the capillaries in our eyes are tiny and the eyes are located above the heart. Deep breathing improves flow of oxygen to the brain, which the eyes are a part of.

Exercise One: Deep Breathing

Here's a helpful breathing exercise to teach you to breathe deeply.

- Breathe in through your nose. Breathe out through the mouth. Place the hands on your belly. As you breathe in, notice your belly rise. As you breathe out, notice your belly flatten.
- Breathe in deeply for a count of three. Hold your breath for a count of four. Breathe out for a count of three.

- As your breathing deepens you can increase the count of the inhalation, holding, and exhale. Repeat this breathing exercise throughout the day when you begin to feel your eyes and body tense.

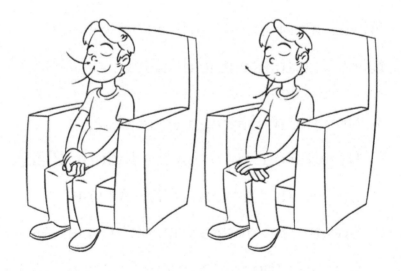

Exercise Two: Lens Flexor

This exercise is from Lisette Scholl's book, *28 Days to Reading without*

Glasses. It will open your breathing, increase circulation and exercise your eyes.

Here's how to do the Lens Flexor.

1. With eyes shut, sit comfortably with both feet flat on the floor.
2. Hold your hands cupped in your lap, one resting on top of the other.
3. Inhale and breathe fully through your nose, maintaining your hands cupped. Stomach should round out.
4. Exhale and flatten out your hands so your palms become parallel to each other. Stomach should contract as you exhale.

Can you feel how the movement coordinates with a flexing sensation in your eyes as your hands open and close?

Stretching

To rest the eyes, you must relax the muscles of the body. When the muscles tense up from mental strain, anxiety and stress, so do the eyeball muscles responsible for acuity of vision. So before actually moving into vision practice, do a quick two minute warm up of your body to relax your arms, neck, and muscles of the upper body.

Here's how.

- Inhale deeply and stretch up from fingers to toes.
- Yawn. Why yawn? Yawning floods the eyes with oxygen rich blood.
- Move your arms circularly from one side to the other, in one direction and then in the other.
- Yawn.
- Tilt your body to one side and then to the other, reaching the opposite arm of the side you are leaning to.
- Yawn.

Movement

"The world moves. Let it move. All objects move if you let them. Do not interfere with this movement, or try to stop it. This cannot be done without an effort which impairs the efficiency of the eye and mind."

Wm H. Bates: *Better Eyesight Magazines*, July 1920

The natural impulse of the eyes is movement. Even when asleep, the eyes are moving during the REM cycles. Lack of motion of the eyes results in staring. Try it. Notice how, when the eyes stop moving by staring, your visual field starts to collapse and vision declines. The less your eyes move, the less they rapidly scan and record details from the environment.

Here are some ways to move your body and, as a result your eyes.

Exercise One: Sway

The sway is a great vision exercise to evoke heightened awareness of the illusion of oppositional movement. The experience is similar to, when you are stationary in a car and another car pulls out. It seems as if the car you are in has started to move. It also has value because when we sway, we allow the body, mind and eyes to relax and the eyes to look rather than see.

Here's how to do it.

1. Stand with legs hip width apart in front of a window.
2. Lower your arms and shoulders and relax the neck
3. Start to swing your body rhythmically from one leg to another. Keep your head still. Feel like a pendulum, swaying back and forth.
4. Look straight ahead but don't try to focus on anything.
5. Notice how when you lean right, near objects move to the left against a distance object, like a car or tree with the converse true as well.
6. Do this 10 times and close your eyes. Imagine the seeming motion of objects and continue to swing the

body.

7. Open your eyes and look at how the objects in your field of vision move.

Exercise Two: Long Swing

Do you remember how you loved swinging on a swing as a child and twirling around? As an adult good chance you enjoy lying in a hammock and swinging gently, or rocking back and forth in a rocking chair. These activities are not only pleasurable but benefit your eyes as well.

You don't need a hammock or swing to move your body to and fro. You can encourage movement through the *Long Swing*.

Benefits of the long swing.

- Increases circulation.
- Limbers the spine to bring flexibility to the body which, in turn, makes the mind more flexible.
- Restores the natural vibratory movement of the eyes
- Helps to achieve eye and mind coordination.
- Increases shifting.
- Switches on your vision and increases clarity as you swing.
- Activates your central vision.
- Encourages lymph flow.

drjohndewitt.com

INTERESTING INFO: *The lymphatic system is the clean-up crew of the body, sweeping out toxins and other unwanted waste products. The human body has twice as much lymphatic fluid as blood but to get it to circulate through the body requires movement as it does not reside in an organ. If your body and eyes don't move much, the lymphatic fluid contained within them doesn't circulate well. Instead, it stagnates within the body and eyes, slowing the visual process. The long swing wakes up your sense of motion helping to move the fluid throughout your body and eyes. This can also be done by using a rebounder which is a* *small trampoline. Easy bouncing causes the lymph to increase circulation in the body.*

Here are guidelines for doing the long swing.

- Remove your glasses and stand up straight.
- Put on music that has the beat to allow you to move your body rhythmically.
- Release to the rhythm and focus on the feeling and movement.
- Keep your eyes soft.
- Notice how the world moves by you, rather than how you move through the world.
- Practice long swings for 15 to 20 minutes at a time and as many times during the day as you can.

HELPFUL HINTS: *Let your body release to the rhythm while keeping your spine straight. This will stimulate the sympathetic nerves and gets your eyes shifting.*

Exercise One

1. Stand comfortably with your feet about a hips width apart.
2. Twist your body 90 degrees to the left and lift your right heel.
3. Twist your body to the right side and lift your left heel.
4. Let your arms fall loosely to your sides and follow your body as it twists.
5. Perform semi-turns with the upper body to the left and right for 10 full rotations.
6. Become aware of everything in the room appearing to slide in the opposite direction that your body is moving – the illusion of oppositional movement. Any time you are moving

in any direction, you can observe it. For instance, when you walk forward the ground appears to be moving backward. If you are nearsighted and the world appears blurry, imagine objects being perfectly clear. Such imaging with your eyes closed will help you see more clearly with your eyes open.

7. Close your eyes and begin slowing down by making your swings shorter and shorter until you return to a still place and feel grounded.

You Don't Need Your Glasses or Contacts

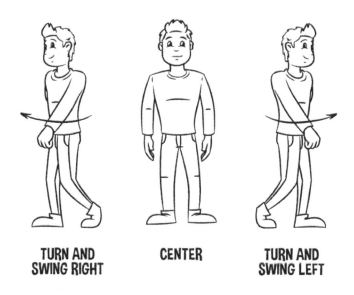

TURN AND SWING RIGHT — CENTER — TURN AND SWING LEFT

HELPFUL TIP: *Make sure you do not:*

- *Twist your torso.*
- *Separate your head from your torso.*
- *Lead from your shoulders.*
- *Try to break out of the swing.*
- *Hold back with the back leg.*

drjohndewitt.com

Exercise Two

1. Perform semi-turns while holding your right arm out, thumb up, as you focus your eyes on your thumb.
2. Repeat with the left arm out, thumb up.
3. Continue moving your entire body fluidly side to side alternating holding out each arm, thumb up and eyes focused on your thumb.

HELPFUL TIP: *If your shoulders are tight and your arms are not falling loosely to your side, hold your hands behind your back instead and alternate while letting them fall loosely to your side and holding them behind your back.*

Exercise Three

Try the long swing with eyes closed and especially if you feel any eye discomfort. This is helpful because seeing is far more mental than physical. By closing your eyes, you will strengthen memory, imagination, visualization and even balance.

To avoid dizziness, try to remember what you saw with your eyes open while swinging. If dizziness continues, open your eyes, stop and focus on one spot until the dizziness subsides.

HELPFUL TIP: *If you cannot perform the long swing, just move your head left to right as if you were shaking your head to say "no." Any swinging motion will break the habit of staring and help loosen the six muscles around each eye to relax eyes and mind.*

How long to swing for?

Do the long swing for 5 to 6 minutes. After 6 minutes, the blood has circulated through the system several times and all the muscles in the body and eyes relax because the nervous system relaxes switches from the sympathetic nervous system, which elicits fight or flight, to the parasympathetic nervous system, which elicits rest and relaxation.

If possible, get into the habit of doing the long swing for 5 to 6 minutes 2 to 3 times a day. Rocking in a rocking chair or swinging in a hammock for 10 to 15 minutes is a comparable experience.

drjohndewitt.com

Exercise Four

Stimulating both sides (hemispheres) of the brain is critical for both clear, close vision and energy (stimulating the left side) and clear far vision and relaxation (stimulating the right side). The Cross-Crawl Exercise is a method to stimulate both sides and accelerate healing of poor vision.

How to do it:
Stand with your shoulders about shoulder width apart. Reach down and across your body with your right hand as you raise your left knee and touch it. Repeat on the opposite side. Look straight ahead in a relaxed manner during this exercise.

drjohndewitt.com

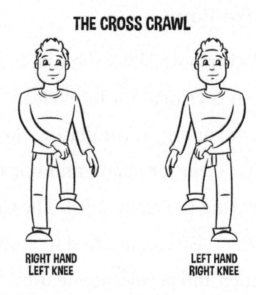

Count to yourself 1, 2, 1, 2 as you perform this exercise or even attempt to do the lazy eights (described later) as you do this, to really over-stimulate the brain.

Notes

Energetic Yawning

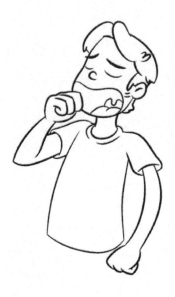

Yawning is one of the best natural things you can do for your eyes. Take your time yawning and fully stretch out those tense jaw muscles (the TMJ), the strongest in the body. Yawning lubricates the eyes, relaxes the muscles of face and mouth, and improves the nerve flow to and from the eyes. Try it now. You might notice your vision a bit clearer?

Blinking

Healthy eyes blink every 2-3 seconds. Do yours? Observe yourself to find out. Good chance that you are not blinking your eyes more than every 20-30 seconds when looking at a screen. Yet, if you deliberately tried *not* to blink for that long it would be hard.

If you want good vision, you need to train yourself to blink frequently and effortlessly. Here's why.

1. Large amounts of dust in the air fall on the surface of eyes.

2. The mind is straining when the eyes are held open.
3. Regular and uninterrupted blinking purifies and lubricates the eyes.
4. Blinking interrupts staring or straining, clearing the "computer screen" and bringing in a fresh view.
5. Blinking relaxes the eyes all day.

HELPFUL HINTS: *If you suffer from dry eyes, do quick, light butterfly blinks several times a day for a minute each time. It should feel wonderfully invigorating.*

Here's how to blink.

- Blink with one eye. Close your eyes for a moment and blink the other eye. In time, switch blinking from one eye to the other without closing the eyes.
- Start the morning with 3 – 5 minutes of blinking to get into the habit. When you notice yourself staring, blink for a minute or two to break up the stare.
- Remind yourself to blink frequently while working at the computer.

Palming

Palming is the Bates trademark relaxation tool and is easy to do. It stimulates the optic nerve and releases the muscles around the eyes, while the warmth and darkness provided by the palms gives your eyes a needed rest, all of which induces deep relaxation. To relax the eyes, you should make it an automatic habit throughout the day.

But don't the eyes rest when we're asleep, you might wonder? Actually no. A good chunk of our sleep is REM or dreaming sleep. During this time, the eyes accommodate to the objects we are "looking at" in our dreams.

When you palm, you will discover something you may not have ever known. When the eyes are truly relaxed, you see blackness like night with eyes closed. This is the mind's feedback that you are truly relaxed. At first, you may see only gray, grainy, cloudy, wavy or glimpse of color. The more you palm, the more relaxed your eyes will become and you will get quicker into this natural state of blackness.

Palming will help you to create a restful state that you maintain by blinking throughout the day. So remember these two magic words: Palming; Blinking.

How to Palm

- Find a comfortable place and position in which to palm, perhaps a comfy armchair, your couch.
- Remove your glasses.
- Lean over from the hips and place your elbows on a desk or table on

something soft like a pillow, whatever position gives you good elbow support or your arms will tire and your shoulders and neck will tense up. Head and neck should be upright as much as possible.

Ways to support the elbows:

- Pillows propped under upper arms
- Blankets
- Table top leaning against a stack of books
- Knees
- Back of chair

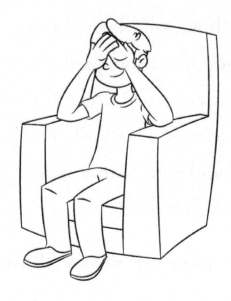

- Shake your hands to warm them up and then rub them together to raise temperature.
- Cup hands slightly, the edges of the palms resting on the bony part around the eyes to shut out as much light as possible. Don't press on the eyes or put any pressure on them. Simply block out all light.

You Don't Need Your Glasses or Contacts

- Close your eyes, relax facial muscles, especially the jaw, and let shoulders get heavy.
- Let your legs relax, with feet flat on the floor when in a chair. Don't cross legs or ankles but keep legs parallel. If need be, lean back in the chair.
- Relax the body completely.

IMPORTANT TIP: *Don't use eye masks as you will lose out on the beneficial energy and warmth only hands can provide.*

- Take in deep, slow breaths (described previously) from your abdomen while palming to encourage relaxation.
- Imagine the color black and see the world get darker and darker as your

eyes relax more and more. Imagining will involve the mind, greatly enhancing relaxation. See the black night sky, or any object or place that reminds you of black color, like black paint, black hair, black piano, black patent leather shoes. The larger the blackness in your field of vision, the more relaxed is your sight.

HELPFUL TIP: For the most restful state while palming, try to stay alert rather than zone off. Listening to relaxing music or thinking out a problem will help you to stay present.

When to Palm

- When eyes feel tired, strained, dry, when your vision gets blurry, or you feel a headache.
- As a regular routine, perhaps to start or end your day.
- After any other vision exercise to rest your eyes and release tension.

IMPORTANT INFO: *The ability to palm for a long period of time and maintain the restful mental state when not palming comes with practice. The more relaxed your vision gets and the less you strain while using your eyes, the less palming you'll need.*

How long to Palm

That answer will vary according to your situation. The more compromised your vision, the longer you will need to palm to relax your eyes and improve your vision. Experiment and see how long it takes to get the results you want. If you suffer from visual processing problems or an eye disease, you will need to palm longer to rest your eyes.

In general, try palming twice a day for **15-30 minutes**. Experiment with different lengths of time and notice how you felt afterwards. This will help to guide you on how long it takes for you to relax your eyes. Palm as needed throughout the day.

drjohndewitt.com

HELPFUL TIP: *The visual field is blacker during palming after movement.*

What to do if you can't relax

If your mind chatters while palming, the following techniques will help you relax and stop your thoughts from racing.

1. Feel your eyes get heavy and sleepy, resting in their sockets. Picture them tilting slightly downward.
2. Imagine a restful scene like watching a sunset or sitting at the ocean on a comfy lounge chair. Remember how peaceful you felt.
3. Observe your breath, breathing in, out, in, out getting longer and longer.
4. Listen to music that relaxes you.
5. Repeat a mantra in your mind.
6. "Write" a love letter to your eyes in your mind, describing how beautiful

and alert they look, and how clearly they can see. Research has shown that imagining something in your mind's eye creates a 70% higher chance of it actually happening. Imagining your eyes with perfect vision will help you to achieve that goal.

Sunning

Do you grab for your sunglasses if the slightest ray of sunshine hits your eyes? Do you find the bright lights in supermarkets and other public venues too bright for you? If so, you are likely light sensitive.

Sensitivity to light is common in the following conditions:

- Macular degeneration
- Second occurrence of cataracts
- Uveitis
- Conjunctivitis
- Corneal abrasion (e.g. through Lasik)
- Viral infection
- Migraine
- Taking certain medications
- Most visual disorders, especially myopia and astigmatism
- Visual processing problems.

Of course, your first tendency is to grab for those sunglasses. But is this the best idea? Not necessarily. Involuntary muscles in the eye, called cilliary muscles, work to open and close the iris to let the proper amount of light into the eye. Overuse of sunglasses lenses can weaken the iris's ability to respond to the environment and increase light sensitivity. *This is likely to happen even more so if you wear tinted glasses (the ones that get darker with more light).* They make the light sensitivity worse and often the refractive error as well, since the amount of available light impacts clarity when vision is not 20/20. In the long run, you will likely need stronger glasses.

A better idea to decrease light sensitivity is the do sunning. One of the core eye relaxation and improvement techniques of the Bates Method, sunning helps get the eyes used to handling light while simultaneously relaxing all the muscles in and around the eye. This happens because when the fovea in the retina is stimulated by light, the light causes the nerve cells of the eye to replenish a pigment in the eye called visual purple.

***INTERESTING INFO:** Sunglasses started out as tools for fighter pilots who, flying high up in the atmosphere had to handle the intense glare of the sun. After World War II, the tinted goggle trend spread throughout the world and now most people in industrialized society wear sunglasses while out in the sun.*

***IMPORTANT INFO:** You need to reverse light sensitivity first before* *being able to improve your myopia or astigmatism.*

Sunning benefits:

- Reduces light sensitivity.
- Strengthens pupillary reflex from the shift from shadow to light when turning the head, which slightly opens and close the pupils.
- Massages the lens capsule through the pupillary reaction, stimulating the photoreceptor cells in the retina without need for sharp focus.
- Release tension and improves blood flow to the neck and shoulder muscles from the warmth of the sunlight and head movement, relaxing the facial muscles.

- Gives you needed vitamin D3 through sun exposure, to absorb the calcium needed to keep bones strong and healthy and boosts the immune system.

TAKE HEED: *If you suffer from macular degeneration or secondary cataracts, do not do sunning.*

How to do basic sunning

1. Go outside and face the sun. You can sit or stand depending on your circumstances at the time.
2. Gently close your eyes and feel the warmth of the bright sunlight on your closed eyelids. Relax your mind with pleasant thoughts or empty it altogether.

3. Inhale slowly and deeply and very slowly turn your head to the left side.
4. Exhale and very slowly turn your head to the right, noticing your right eye now being in the shade and your left eye receiving more light and warmth. Notice the vibrant light in the center when both eyes get an equal amount of light. You may see sunspots of a rosy or purple light, especially if your eyes are not used to light because visual purple is depleted by light and replenished by darkness (palming).
5. Let the breath initiate the turns of the head.
6. Continue going back and forth, as if you were saying "no," turning your

head sideways as far as your neck allows you.

HELPFUL HINT: *If your chin doesn't go all the way to the shoulder for a 180 degree head turn, do not force it. With daily sunning, your tight neck and shoulder muscles will relax and release tension, and in turn improve blood flow to the brain and help you to improve your vision. Tight neck and shoulder muscles are a big contributor to tension in the eyes and vision problems. To help with neck tension, try doing a few "yes" movements with your head, tilting the head slightly back as you inhale and moving the chin toward your chest as you exhale.*

Advanced sunning techniques

Once your eyes get accustomed to sunning, you can deepen the experience by doing the following:

- When head is turned to the sides, open your eyes and blink rapidly.

- Hold your hands in front of your eyes with fingers spread and rapidly move them up and down with eyes open, and blink rapidly. The fingers provide a filter that allows some sun to enter the eyes without being too strong. This is the technique I utilized to correct my own vision.

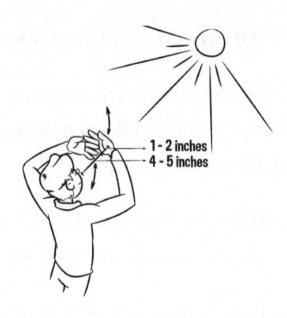

TAKE HEED: *Ultraviolet light from the sun can cause cataract and macular degeneration. If you have an eye condition that requires you to wear sunglasses to keep out ultraviolet light, get the lightest tint you can find.*

How long to sun for

Sun for five to ten minutes or however long you can.

IMPORTANT INFO: *Sunning accustoms your eyes to light and palming accustoms your eyes to dark.* Sunning should always be followed by palming to build up the ability of the eyes to replenish visual purple. Never sun without palming; however, **you can palm without sunning.**

When to sun

Sun in the early morning or late afternoon hours when the sun is lowest if you are used to wearing sunglasses when outside. Otherwise any time of day is fine. You can sun anywhere, and anytime when you are out in the sun.

If you find facing the sun with closed eyes too strong even in with the morning or late afternoon sun, practice on an overcast day or stand with your back to the sun until you feel comfortable enough to face the sun.

INTERESTING INFO: *Your eyes are light receptors constructed to respond to light. Good vision is a highly developed sense of light perception, and people and animals living in bright light have the keenest eyesight.*

What to do after sunning

Blink:

Follow sunning with 5 minutes of blinking into the light. The light relaxes your eyes and mind, and the heat soothes tight muscles.

Palm:

After blinking, palm for ideally twice as long as you did sunning. If you don't have the time, sun until images or colors have faded and your visual field with eyes closed is dark again.

Both palming and sunning keep the eyes young and flexible and allow you to take in natural full spectrum sunlight with ease. This makes both the most important things you can do to eliminate light sensitivity and improve vision.

HELPFUL HINT: *Should your eyes get watery, itchy or start to twitch, it's usually a symptom of the intense strain you're carrying in your eyes. Continue to do the sunning in a relaxed way, and it will slowly melt that tension away. Maybe do it for shorter periods or only with the morning or evening sun until the worst strain is released. I did sunning for about 20 seconds to start and had great results.*

HELPFUL TIP: *If the real sun is not shining or if you live in a part of the world where you get little sun, especially in winter, you can "sun" inside, using a high wattage white infrared lamp, like the OTT lamp.*

Notes

Pinhole Glasses

Try this. Take off your glasses and create a pinhole with your hand by bending your finger to create a small pinhole between the skin folds. Notice how clear your vision becomes without any corrective lenses. Now hold the pinhole in front of your eye, and notice how much more in focus everything is that you're looking at.

Pinhole glasses are glasses with many small holes in the lenses.

You Don't Need Your Glasses or Contacts

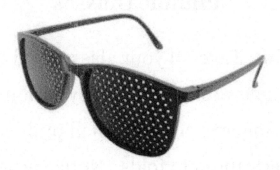

An affordable alternative to prescription eyeglasses for some, they are comprised of precision-manufactured lightweight perforated plastic lenses, inset into standard metal or plastic eyeglass frames.

They work by reducing the amount of light entering the eye allowing your eyes to relax. In a healthy eye, light rays are focused into a single point on the light sensitive retina located at the back of the eyeball. Less healthy eyes focus light rays in front of or behind the retina, casting a blurred circle on the retina. The minute pinholes on the surface of the plastic lenses allow a narrower beam of light through to the eye lens with a greater depth of field. The narrow beam casts a smaller blur circle on the retina, improving vision. Since the pinholes allow only direct and coherent light rays to pass through into the eye, they are ideal for those with refractive eye disorders, seniors and computer users.

Pinhole glasses can "improve" vision and allow you to read or see with less blur, but only while worn.

Here are the many benefits of pinhole glasses.

- Improved visual clarity and resolution.
- Increased apparent object brightness, especially helpful for those who struggle with vision in low-light situations.
- See clearly at all distances.
- Less stressful on the eyes.
- One pair covers seeing near and far.
- Lightweight and durable.
- Affordable (they typically run around $15 to $20).

Alternate Eye Movements

This simple exercise stretches the eye muscles to give them a warm up before further practice. You can do this exercise anytime, and in any place.

- With eyes open, move your eyes open up to down while keeping your head still.
- Move your eyes left to right and vice versa, keeping your head still.
- Repeat whole procedure several times.
- Move your eyes diagonally from bottom-left to top right and vice versa.
- Move your eyes in a circle, clockwise and counter-clockwise several times.
- Repeat whole sequence with eyes shut.

As you can see from the illustration, the eye movements accord with sensory synesthesia. This is how law enforcement can determine if a person is lying or being truthful. Up and to the left is recalling a memory, up and to the right, as you observe them, shows they are making the story up.

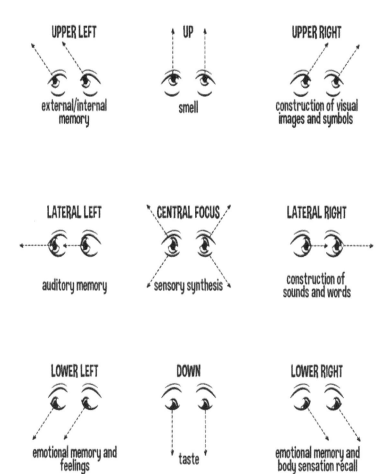

Lazy Eights

This simple exercise packs a punch.

- It integrates both hemispheres of the brain.
- Relaxes the muscles of the hand and arm.
- Supports eye movement.
- Encourages eye-hand coordination.

Here's how to do it.

Track the sign of eternity or the figure eight with your the dominant hand, the eyes following. Start by moving your eyes from center to the left and top. Repeat the same exercise by making a lazy eight with your thumb, with your eyes following.

You Don't Need Your Glasses or Contacts

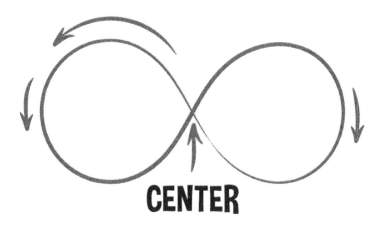

CENTER

Notes

Central Fixation

The clearest point of our field of vision should be the one point we are looking at. This is *central fixation*. Anything in the periphery will not be as clear. Any attempt to bring everything in the entire visual field into focus creates strain and decreased vision.

These central fixation exercises will help reawaken the *fovea centralis* and restore the eye to its normal rapid speed of 60 to 70 vibrations per second. Located in the back of the retina, the fovea centralis, or central pit is your center of sight that allows you to see fine details and colors. It is filled with cones stimulated and activated by movement.

When you stare, your center of sight does not get stimulated. As a result, you may experience more blur. The cones see color and the other specialized receptors, rods, see black and white (used in dim lighting).

HELPFUL HINT: *One of the best ways to break the stare and foster eye movement is through deep, rhythmic breathing along with regular light blinking.*

Here are some ways to practice central fixation.

Exercise One: Tibetan Wheel

Gaze at the diagram of the Tibetan Wheel.

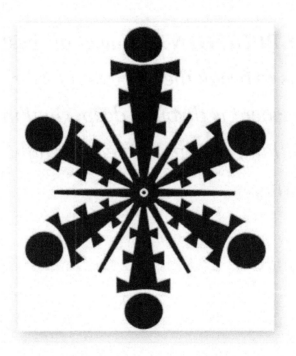

Information from the following website:
http://integraleyesight.com/batesmethod/centralization/Fusion

drjohndewitt.com

1. Start at the top circle. Note how much clearer, blacker and more distinct it is than the other circles. Work your way around, maintaining focus on the point you are looking at.
2. After scanning the outside, make your way further in toward the center until you reach the tiny black dot in the very center. Close your eyes and imagine this tiny black dot.
3. As you go through your day and your eyes focus in on something, imagine this tiny black dot. Doing so will help you to stop trying to see everything clearly at once and instead to see everything in small parts that make up one clear whole.

Exercise 2: Snellen Chart

20/200	**E**	20 FT / 6 1M **1**
20/100	**F P**	100 FT / 6 1M **2**
20/70	**T O Z**	70 FT / 6 1M **3**
20/50	**L P E D**	50 FT / 6 1M **4**
20/40	**P E C F D**	40 FT / 6 1M **5**
20/30	E D F C Z P	30 FT / 6 1M **6**
20/25	F E L O P Z D	25 FT / 6 1M **7**
20/20	D E F P O T E C	20 FT / 6 1M **8**
20/15	L E F O D P C T	15 FT / 6 1M **9**
20/13	F D P L T C E O	13 FT / 6 1M **10**

drjohndewitt.com

1. Look at the top end of the largest letter on the chart. You should see its bottom part worse than the top end and the top end with the greatest visual acuity.
2. When you find the point of greatest acuity, move your sight smoothly downwards and across the letters of the sharpest area your eyes see.
3. Repeat six times.

Exercise Three: Domino Chart

This exercise is designed to make the eyes move in as many different directions as possible.

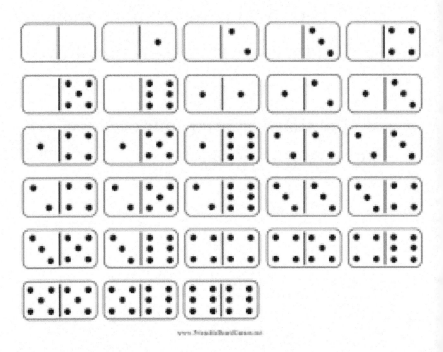

From www.printableboardgames.net

1. Place the chart in front of you so you don't have to strain to see the dominoes.
2. Move your eyes through the consecutive rows of cubes, from left to right and then again to the left but a row below. Continue until you reach the bottom row. Focus not on the dominoes but on smooth eye movement.
3. Now do the same but move through the vertical columns until you reach the last one.
4. Next, move your eyes obliquely, upwards and a cube down through the dominoes.

Exercise Four: Edging

Edging is a technique of motion and central fixation. It involves brushing around the outline of shapes with your nose by letting your eyes follow the "brush" as if there was a paintbrush on the end of the nose. The key is to maintain a relaxed sense of the points flowing into your mind while allowing your attention to move around the outline noticing detail. For close vision, close your eyes and use your finger to draw on a point between the eyes. The mind follows the movement of the fingers.

Here's how to do it.

drjohndewitt.com

You Don't Need Your Glasses or Contacts

1. Remove your glasses and relax.
2. Find a line in your environment at a comfortable distance so you do not strain to see it. It can be the line where a wall joins the ceiling or floor, the edge of a table, door, or other piece of furniture in the room.
3. Feel your feet on the floor, close your eyes, and relax.
4. Open your eyes and move your head and follow your nose along the line noticing every point as you go and that the point you are on is the point you see best.
5. When you get good at this, add motion.

HELPFUL TIP: *Don't jump over points in a line but try to maintain a smooth motion with your eyes and head.*

HELPFUL TIP: *If you have worn or currently wear glasses, you probably have an unconscious mental habit of straining and you might strain when edging. If so, practice for short periods only, palm before and after edging, and keep an awareness of motion and see one part best while you practice.*

Exercise Five: Mandala

Follow a mandala with your nose.

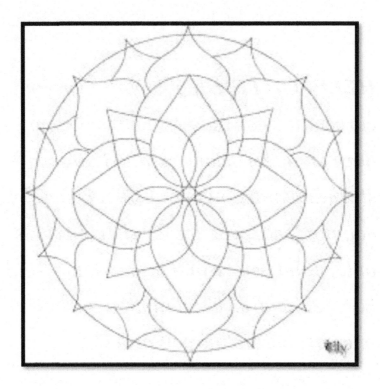

Notes

Fusion

To see clearly, both eyes must fix or converge on the same object at the same time. This requires the eyes to work together as a team. Up close, the eyes must converge by turning inward. At a distance, the eyes must diverge, or turn back out. Strain or tension in one or more of the eye muscles prevents the eyes from working together as team to focus on the same point.

A great exercise to practice fusion or conversion is by using a rope or a string.

Here's how:

- Using a 10-foot string, thread 15 brightly colored beads of varying colors through the rope at six-inch intervals.
- Tie the end of the string to a doorknob or distant object.
- Sit comfortably in a chair, or stand far enough so that you can pull the string taught. Hold it near the tip of the nose so that the eyes gaze across its length.

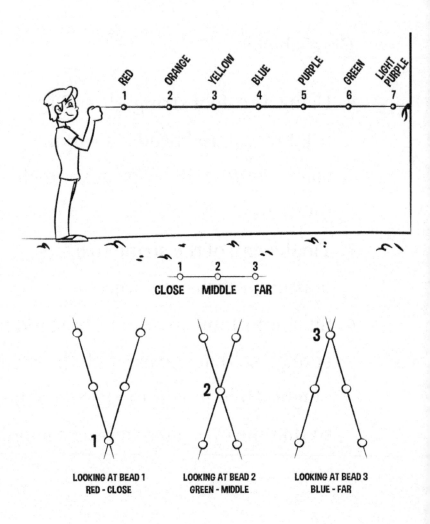

Exercise 1

1. Hold the loose end to the tip of your nose and pull the string tight.
2. Breathing deeply, look with both eyes at the first bead nearest the nose for a few seconds and try to bring it into focus. With normal vision, you should see two lines feeding into the hole making the shape of the letter V. You see two lines because your brain registers the two images coming from your two eyes and combines them at the hole in the bead.

HELPFUL TIPS: *If you have constant or short-distance exotropia, you will only see one line. If this happens, relax your gaze by blinking slowly a couple of times and concentrate on using both eyes to look at the bead. If this doesn't work, try covering one eye, then the other. This will let you know which eye needs training to see both lines.*

3. Once the two eyes converge, hold your vision for 10 seconds.
4. Repeat while focusing on the second and then the third beads and down the line. When focusing anywhere along the middle, the rope should make the shape of the letter X. When focusing on the doorknob, the rope should make the shape of the letter A, or an upside down V.
5. Repeat the series five times, if you can.

Exercise 2:

1. Track the eyes up and down the rope from nose to doorknob. If you struggle, cover one eye.

2. Reverse to move back toward the face until all beads have been focused on.

Exercise 3

1. Look at the closest bead and then the farthest bead, attempting to focus.
2. Look at the second bead, then the farthest again, then the third and so forth, up and down the string, pausing on each to attempt to focus.

Notes

Eye Oblique Muscle Stretch

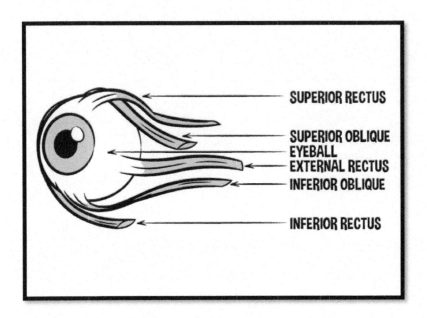

This exercise will relax the eye oblique muscles used to change the eye optical length. *Don't skip this exercise as the eye oblique muscles are responsible for proper and acute vision.*

Here's how to do it.

You Don't Need Your Glasses or Contacts

1. Using a pencil or your thumb move it slowly from down, near the body and move it towards the tip of the nose.
2. Look at the tip of your finger until it touches the nose and your eyes turn also to that point (near the nose you may see two thumbs).
3. Move horizontally to the right still looking at the finger as it is moving. Stop briefly and move back toward the nose.
4. Repeat moving horizontally to the left.
5. When moving to a particular direction, breathe in, stop for 1-2 seconds, exhale when moving towards the nose to relax the muscles.

drjohndewitt.com

Near / Far Exercise

This exercise will teach you to fully contract and relax the eyes. This will train the muscles to become stronger and more efficient at their job.

Here's how to do it.

1. Remove your glasses.
2. Look at an object in the distance, like a tree with a soft gaze, without any strain.
3. Look at an object between you and the furthest object, for instance the car in front of you.
4. Hold up your finger as close to your nose as possible without strain and look at it.

5. Shift your focus from far to middle to near continuously, i.e. tree, car, finger.

6. Try to do this 10 times.

Eye-Mind Connection

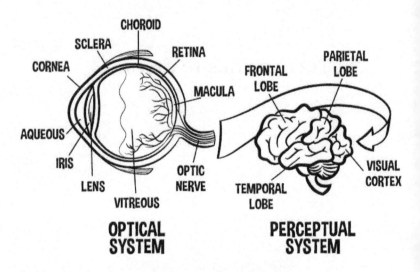

VISUAL SYSTEM

Vision is 90% mental and 10% physical. The eyes simply take in light, while the mind interprets the electrical impulses sent from the retina through the optic nerve to the visual cortex in the back of the brain. For this reason, much of the Bates Method is geared toward rebuilding the connection between mind and body we all once had.

How do you create an eye-mind coordination? You need to focus the eyes, your attention and the mind all on the same thing at the same time. In other words, you need to be present. If you are thinking about checking your emails when you are palming, you are not present and focused and the mind is in charge and you are less likely to have relaxed eyes that see black. Here are some exercises to help you re-establish the mind-body connection from the helpful website www.bateseyeexercises.com.

Visualization

When we visualize, our eyes are actively accommodating what the mind is trying to see. Over time, visualization, will help us learn to relax the eyes more and improve the power and acuity of sight.

For best results, practice these exercises while palming.

Exercise 1: Ship sailing out

1. Sit in a comfortable chair. Relax and close your eyes.
2. Imagine standing on the pier in front of a large passenger ship.
3. You can see men and women, young and old talking, children running back and forth, men and women in

You Don't Need Your Glasses or Contacts

uniform carrying trays. Some are standing looking out at the ocean, or at the land, while others stroll through the decks.

4. Slowly, the large ship sets sail and you are seeing less and less details on the decks. The windows and human silhouettes are smaller and smaller. The sea surrounds the ship more and more. The sun is shining. The ship is getting smaller and smaller and you can't make out any passengers. Finally, the ship is just a dot on the horizon.

Now do this exercise.

1. Reverse the course of events and first see the ship as a dot that sails to shore

and becomes more and more detailed. Slowly, you begin to see people on the decks, tables and portholes. Continue this imaginary scene until the ship reaches the port and you are standing next to it.
2. Repeat the moving away and coming of the ship in your mind several times. Slowly, speed up this process.

By continuing to imagine the ship sailing away and coming nearer, your eyes are moving in and out, helping the muscles and refraction of the eyeball. Also notice how the exercise has helped you relax.

Exercise 2: Runners on the track

1. Sit in a comfortable chair. Relax and close your eyes.
2. Imagine that you are standing at the start line of the race on a large track.
3. You see several athletes hunched down at the start line. Look at them closely and notice the details in their outfit, body, or behavior.
4. Imagine that the race begins and you are watching how the runners are running even further, moving away from you and around the track. As the runners move away, you can see less and less details. Finally, they become small dots in the farthest location from you.

5. Now see the athletes running on the track coming near to the finish line and you. You see more and more details of the runners, their outfits, facial expression, body characteristics. Finally they reach the finish line where you are standing.
6. Practice them moving away and coming nearer in your mind several times. Slowly speed it up.

With eyes closed, this exercise has a great benefit for the eye muscles and refraction of the eyeball.

Notes

Analytic Vision

As Bates continually impressed upon us, an immobilized eyeball hinders vision and creates watery and dim sight, and inability to see normally. Proper vision entails minimal and permanent eye movement. You see this in observing people with normal sight, who maintain their eyes such that they move unconsciously constantly from one point of an object to another with minimum effort.

This analytic vision exercise is designed to help you to acquire minimum and constant eye movement. At first, these actions will be conscious but over time they will become automatic and unconscious and you will look freely and without effort.

Here's what to do.

1. When looking at something, for instance a building, try to draw with your eyes the external contours of a building, across the gutter, roof and ground.
2. Look at the windows, door, banister, roof while trying to draw with your eyes the external edges.

3. Move quickly from one element to another, choosing different types and directions of eye movement without seeing these parts of a building acutely.
4. Blink freely to ensure that your eyes are moistened and rested.
5. Now look at the building as a whole. Does it seem clearer to you?

Notes

Nutrition

Optimal vision is not only determined by the extraocular muscles of the eye. These exercises and stretches have helped with that but now we must focus on the whole body. The foods we eat are another piece of this puzzle and play a large role in healing as well.

Vitamin A

Remember that in order to be able to see, our specialized cells (rods and cones) located in the retina must need to function well. After the light hits these receptors they get bleached, these visual pigments need to regenerate in order to keep doing what they need to do. Vitamin A helps that regeneration process.

Vitamin C

Vitamin C strengthens the immune system to protect the body from pathogens. It has the same effect on the eyes. Vitamin C acts as an antioxidant that protects the cells in the eyes from damage caused by harmful allergens from the environment. It also promotes healing which helps maintain a healthy cornea and overall eye vitality.

Vitamin E:

Vitamin E is also important for better vision. It helps in the synthesis of red blood cells which is critical for eye health. Vitamin E is most beneficial to the eyes as it can protect our visual organs from free radicals which abound in the environment.

Antioxidants:

Natural antioxidants beta-carotene, zeaxanthin and lutein can also help your vision. These antioxidants may sound alien for some but these powerhouses are now commonly incorporated in all kinds of health products from bath soaps to nutritional supplements. In the eyes, they protect the macula, which is located in the middle of the eye ball, from sun damage. Proper antioxidant intake helps ensure that you are taking the necessary steps to slow down age-related macular degeneration.

DHA, Omega-3s:

DHA from fish oils can help strengthen your cell membranes and it can provide structural support for your eyes and boosts your entire eye health. Omega 3s are also a natural anti-inflammatory and help to regenerate the cartilage of the joints. They are another nutrient that helps prevent macular degeneration.

Zinc:

Zinc is a mineral that is necessary for cell division and cell division is a process necessary for healing and growth. This helps the "repigmentation" of the rods and cones in the retina of the eyes.

20 Surprising Foods to Promote Eye Health

When you were younger, you were probably told countless times that some orange colored foods, specifically carrots, promote healthy eyes. While you may think that your parents' efforts to protect your vision were a cover up to get you to eat all your vegetables, there's some truth in what they were saying. These orange foods are more than meets the eye (no pun intended); they contain large amounts of Beta-carotene, a form of vitamin A, which is responsible for giving these orange foods their bright color. Beta-carotene is known to help restore and maintain the health of the retina, which in turn helps your eyes to function properly.

Carrots are the obvious food for better eyesight, even our parents knew this, but keeping your eyes healthy through your diet doesn't just rely on beta-carotene alone. There are a number of other beneficial vitamins and minerals that are just as important for healthy eyes.

At the end of the day, there's some truth in the old adage 'You are what you eat!' Eating healthily on a daily basis is essential for your overall health, especially your eyes' health. Here are some of the most powerful foods you should be including in your diet to help promote healthy eyes and vision.

Leafy Greens

Leafy greens are also probably one of the food groups your parents were trying to get you to eat more of when you were younger, and again they're right, but probably not for the same reasons they were advocating. Leafy greens that include kale, spinach, collard, lettuce, broccoli, and cabbage are jam-packed with a whole lot of zeaxanthin and lutein, two powerful antioxidants that have been proven to help reduce the risk of degeneration of the eye and cataracts later on in life.

Eggs

It doesn't matter if they're boiled, scrambled, fried or in an omelet, eggs are an excellent source of nutrition for your eyes. The yolk of the egg is especially powerful as it contains a good amount of lutein, zeaxanthin, and zinc. Like your leafy greens, the egg yolk can help maintain your eyes' health as you grow older, and essentially it can help fight cataracts. The yolk of an egg also contains a great source of natural vitamin D, which over the years has been proven to help reduce the risk of developing ARMD (age-related macular degeneration), which results in vision loss later on in life.

Citrus fruits

Oranges, lemons, limes, and grapefruit are all full of vitamin C. Vitamin C is superior to most other vitamins, and it's one of the best forms of antioxidants. Vitamin C is known to form and maintain your body's connective tissues, which also includes the collagen found in your eye's cornea. Eating more citrus fruit will help protect your eyes from trauma to the eyes and prevent them from being damaged.

Seeds and nuts

Seeds and nuts may be your favorite snack food, but they're also more beneficial than this, they're excellent sources of vitamins C and E. When combined, these vitamins work together to help keep your body's tissues strong and healthy which is essential for healthy eyes as the dense outer layer of the eye is made up of tissues. Eat more sunflower seeds, chia seeds, flaxseeds, almonds, peanuts, and pecans.

Wild Blueberries

If there were a super fruit, it would surely be the blueberry. It is unbelievable how one little fruit can contain so much goodness. This humble berry is in fact one of the foods with the highest amounts of antioxidants. While the blueberry is beneficial in many ways and tackles a number of health concerns, it's especially beneficial when it comes to maintaining your eyes' health. Blueberries contain high doses of vitamin C, which help fight the free radicals responsible for damaging your eyes and causing eye disease. Getting more vitamin C in your diet will help reduce any intraocular pressure on the eye, meaning you'll have less of a chance of developing glaucoma later on in life, which is the second leading cause of blindness in adults in the US. Why wild, organic blueberries? They have been shown to have higher levels of these life saving nutrients.

Sweet Potatoes

If you're not already substituting potatoes with sweet potatoes, this may make you think again. Sweet potatoes aren't only for Thanksgiving; this delicious and understated vegetable is packed with vitamin A, a powerful antioxidant. Vitamin A is responsible for protecting your eyes against any nasty free radicals that can harm your eyes. Vitamin A is particularly helpful by reducing eye inflammation and dry eyes, which are two things that, if left untreated, could lead to some more serious eye problems later on down the road.

Fatty Fish

If you don't eat much fish, you might want to reconsider your diet. Fatty fish in particular is rich in DHA, a special fatty acid that's also found in your eye's retina. Research shows that low levels of DHA in the eye can lead to dry eyes and dry eye syndrome. So, if you want to avoid refractive surgery in the future, eat more wild salmon, mackerel, tuna, trout, and anchovies. If you're one of these people who don't like fish, it's essential to take capsules containing omega-3 essential fatty acid to prevent dryness of the eyes.

Whole Grains

Whole grains have always been promoted as the 'healthy' food, but we're never really told why. A diet that has a low glycemic index (GI) will dramatically reduce your risk of developing any eye condition related to ageing such as macular degeneration. Additionally, whole grains contain an impressive amount of vitamin E, niacin and zinc, which together will help with you overall eye health. Ditch the refined carbs in your diet such as white breads and pasta and opt for brown rice, oats, whole-wheat breads, and quinoa instead.

Legumes

Legumes are powerful sources of nutrition, and they provide your body with an excellent dose of zinc and bioflavonoids, which help protect the eye's retina. It also reduces the risk of developing any age-related eye condition in the future such as macular degeneration and cataracts. Countries in the Middle East and the Mediterranean, where diets are high in lentils, haricot beans, kidney beans, and black-eyed peas, have lower rates of cataracts than countries that diets don't include such high amount of legumes.

Grass Fed Beef

Dismiss any information that tells you beef is unhealthy. When eaten in moderation, beef can boost your health ten-fold, especially your eye health. Always opt for the leaner, grass fed versions, but beef in general has high amounts of zinc. Zinc works together with vitamin A, a vitamin essential for eye health. Zinc helps assist the absorption of vitamin A, so essentially vitamin A is useless without zinc. With the combination of vitamin A and zinc, you'll help reduce the risk of any age-related eye conditions, such as macular degeneration.

Coconut Milk

Coconut milk is full of amazingly helpful medium chain triglycerides that has a laundry list of beneficial effects including:

1. An additional energy source for brain function which includes the visual center.

2. Antimicrobial effects fighting of these viruses:
- HIV
- measles
- herpes simplex (HSV-1)
- vesicular stomatitis virus
- visna virus
- cytomegalovirus (CMV)

3. All natural SunScreen

These are just a few of the amazing characteristics of coconut, coconut oil and coconut milk.

Tomatoes

Tomatoes may just be that simple red

fruit you find in your salad, but these fruits are packed with carotenoids, which are responsible for the tomato's bright red color. Lycopene, which is one of the important carotenoids in tomatoes, helps promote the eyes' ocular tissues and helps reduce any light-induced damage to the eye's retina.

Olive Oil

Olive oil is not just a dressing for your salad or a healthy way of frying it's also a great way to help protect your eyes' health. When you consciously follow a diet that has a low amount of trans and saturated fats, you'll reduce the risk of contracting retina diseases. Research also shows it helps reduce the risk of ARMD by a whopping

48%. If you're buying olive oil, make sure you go for the extra virgin version as this contains more antioxidants.

Non-GMO Corn

If you're a corn lover, you're in luck. Corn has high amounts of lutein and zeaxanthin, and only ½ a cup of boiled corn contains 1.8g of healthy pigments per serving. The pigments that are found in corn are also naturally occurring in the eye, but when ARMD sets in, these pigments are lost. When you eat more foods that contain such rich pigments, you significantly reduce the risk of losing your eyes' natural pigments.

Pistachios

Although pistachios fall into the category of nuts, they're worthy of their own mention as they contain high amounts of zeaxanthin and lutein, which help restore the retina and ward off ARMD. Not only are they high in these antioxidants, they also contain high amounts of vitamin E and eating pistachios can reduce the risk of developing cataracts and other age-related eye diseases. If this isn't enough, pistachios also contain mono and polyunsaturated fats that help accelerate the absorption of carotenoids, thus making the pistachio one of the healthiest snacks for your eyes.

Strawberries

Who doesn't love this tasty summer fruit? Not only are strawberries the perfect partner for cream and ice cream they also contain a number of beneficial nutrients to help you reach optimal eye health and sight. Strawberries have high amounts of vitamin C, which will help you fight and reduce inflammation of the eyes. It doesn't matter whether the inflammation is naturally occurring or self-inflicted from wearing makeup or your contacts too long, strawberries help reduce it. These red succulent berries also contain a variety of powerful antioxidants that will help your body defend your eyes when it comes to eye infections, dryness, and macular degeneration. All it takes is a cup of strawberries a day to help eliminate or prevent eye problems.

Avocado

Toss it in a salad, spread it on toast or eat whole, when eaten raw, avocado provides your body with vitamins B6, C and E, all of which are essential for healthy eyesight. Avocado also helps reduce your stress levels, and while it's not directly related to your eyesight, stress has been proven to be one of the causes of vision loss.

Peppers

No matter what form or color your

peppers come in, they're all beneficial to your eyes. Make eating all kinds of peppers of all colors a routine as they're one of the best sources of vitamins A and C. Peppers cooked or raw contain beta-carotene, vitamin B6, lutein, lycopene, and zeaxanthin, all of which help improve your eyesight.

Dark Chocolate

Rich in antioxidants, dark chocolate does wonders for your eyes. It is made up of powerful antioxidants like flavonols, which are known to enhance the blood flow to the eye's retina, thus helping your eyes to see evenly when the light is low.

Tea and Coffee

Tea and coffee may be surprising addition to the list to promote eye health, but research shows that drinking tea and coffee can assist in preventing macular degeneration, cataracts and dry eyes. Coffee and tea also stops the growth of new blood vessels towards the back of the eyes, which can cause vision loss if there's a buildup over time.

Your eyes are a gift, but more often than not we take them and our sight for granted. Our eyes are busy working tirelessly throughout the day, and you've just got to think about what they get exposed to on a daily basis. TV, cell phones, computers, newspapers, books, and signs to name but a few are some of things we expose our eyes to. Because we use our eyes so much without even realizing it, we're more vulnerable to common eye problems such as distorted vision, poor eyesight, and cataracts. As soon as you begin to develop problems with your eyes, your world can change depending on how severe the problem is. But with the right diet and taking precautions, you can do your part and help preserve your eyes and sight for years to come.

Notes

Chiropractic Care and your Vision – What's the Connection?

Your eyes and vision are important. They're so important that we often greatly underestimate what they can do. It's interesting that various parts of the body are interconnected, and if one area functions inadequately, it's quite possible this would effect other areas of the body as well. What's even more interesting is the unique relationship between your vision and chiropractic care, but then again it's not really surprising considering that your body's nervous system is the power hub which controls and coordinates every single function in your body, which also includes your vision.

Your optic nerve is part of your body's nervous system, which is responsible for supplying a lot of information to the brain. If there's any disruption of any kind to your body's nerve communication, the input, communication and functioning will be abnormal.

Because everything in your body is connected, something seemingly normal such as a spinal misalignment, which is also known as subluxation, can cause huge disruptions to your body's central nervous system. This is when your chiropractor will step in; it's their job to locate such problems and fix them before they become more serious. And this is also the reason why your chiropractor may be able to pinpoint the cause of some of your vision problems better than your ophthalmologist. Traditionally, chiropractic care isn't typically seen as a remedy or a cure for blindness or other vision impairments. However, if you talk with your chiropractor, they're likely to tell you that they've experienced a number of instances where their chiropractic patients' vision improved after undergoing chiropractic adjustments.

Studies show there's a relationship between chiropractic care and an improvement in eyesight and there have been a number of different known cases of this occurring. One particular case involved a young girl, who had impaired vision from the bilateral concentric narrowing of her visual fields. Such a condition was once considered to be more permanent, but after visiting her chiropractor for just one spinal adjustment, her vision was restored back to normal.

The young girl went for one whole year without suffering from any vision problems after her standard spinal adjustment procedure until one day she was suddenly hit on the head by a flying ball. Being hit in the head caused her

vision problems to return once more. After having another spinal adjustment, her sight was once again restored.
The abovementioned case is even more proof that there's a connection before chiropractic care and vision. When the head receives a hit or even just a slight knock, it can result in problems of the neck and spine, and in some cases it can even alter the spine's curvature. When the cervical spine is damaged, it can lead to a number of different nervous system problems, which naturally includes vision problems.

Another case in point is a 62-year-old male. He had been suffering from monocular vision problems coupled with ongoing headaches and a neck strain. Initially, it was believed that he was just experiencing vision problems that come with age, however after a fundoscopic examination, doctors failed to find any abnormalities in his optic nerve or retina. After having visited a chiropractor for a period of a week to receive spinal manipulative therapy, his headaches, neck strain and vision problems disappeared.

Other vision problems that chiropractic care can help improve or restore are oculomotor functioning, visual acuity, pupillary size, and intraocular pressure. So, how does chiropractic care help?

The spine and the optic nerve's blood supply are directly connected to the vertebral artery's closeness to the cervical spine. In simpler terms, the eye's blood supply is closely connected to your cervical spine's health and positioning.

Chiropractic care is not a direct treatment for vision impairments and problems, but when the spine is aligned properly in a number of patients, they have experienced better vision. Today, some chiropractors focus on just the spine's health, however, many more are moving towards the idea of spine alignment being connected to a person's overall health.

drjohndewitt.com

Notes

SUMMING UP

Through the Bates Method, you can improve vision for short sight, long sight, astigmatism, old-age sight, squint, 'lazy' eye, and even structural diseases such as macular degeneration.

The secret is to use the eyes normally and, more importantly, to relax them.

It's as simple as that.

Bates Exercises...Overview

Relaxation

Breathing: Deep breathing improves flow of oxygen to the brain which the eyes are a part of. Three exercises to help you to learn to breathe more deeply are: Deep Breathing and Lens Flexor.

Stretching: To rest the eyes, you must relax the muscles of the body. When the muscles tense up from mental strain, anxiety and stress, so do the eyeball muscles responsible for acuity of vision. So before actually moving into vision practice, do a quick two minute warm up of your body to relax your arms, neck, and muscles of the upper body.

drjohndewitt.com

Movement:

The natural impulse of the eyes is movement. Even when asleep, the eyes are moving during the REM cycles. Lack of motion of the eyes results in staring. Some exercises that will help you move your body and as a result your eyes are the sway and the long swing.

Energetic Yawning: Yawning is one of the best natural things you can do for your eyes. It lubricates the eyes, relaxes the muscles of face and mouth, and improves the nervous system to and from the eyes.

Blinking: Healthy eyes blink every 2-3 seconds. It's important to get into the habit of blinking.

Palming: Palming is the Bates trademark relaxation tool and is easy to do. It stimulates the optic nerve and releases the muscles around the eyes, while the warmth and darkness provided by the palms gives your eyes a needed rest, all of which induces deep relaxation. The more you palm, the more relaxed your eyes will become and you will get quicker into this natural state of blackness. For this reason, palming should become an automatic habit throughout the day.

Sunning: Sunning is a great exercise to help relieve light sensitivity. It does so by getting the eyes used to handling light while simultaneously relaxing all the muscles in and around the eye.

Pinhole Glasses: Pinhole glasses are glasses with many small holes in the lenses. They work by reducing the amount of light entering the eye allowing your eyes to relax. Pinhole glasses can "improve" vision and allow you to read or see with less blur, but only while worn.

Alternate Eye Movements: This simple exercise stretches the eye muscles to give them a warm up before further practice. You can do this exercise anytime, and in any place.

Lazy Eights

Track the sign of eternity or the figure eight with your dominant hand, the eyes following. Start by moving your eyes from center to the left and top. Repeat the same exercise by making a lazy eight with your thumb, with your eyes following.

Central Fixation

The clearest point of our field of vision should be the one point we are looking at. This is central fixation. Any attempt to bring everything in the entire visual field into focus creates strain and decreased vision. Central fixation exercises will help reawaken the fovea centralis, our center pit and restore the eye to its normal rapid speed of 60 to 70 vibrations per second. Exercises to practice central fixation include: Tibetan Wheel, Snellen Chart, Domino chart, Edging and following a Mandala with your nose.

Fusion

To see clearly, both eyes must fix or converge on the same object at the same time. This requires the eyes to work together as a team. Up close, the eyes must converge by turning inward. At a distance, the eyes must diverge, or turn back out. Strain or tension in one or more of the eye muscles prevents the eyes from working together as team to focus on the same point. A great exercise to practice fusion or conversion is by using a rope or a string.

Eye Oblique Muscle Stretch

This exercise will relax the eye oblique muscles used to change the eye optical length.

Near / Far

This exercise will teach you to fully contract and relaxing the eyes. This will train the muscles to become stronger and more efficient at its job.

Eye-Mind Connection

Vision is 90% mental and 10% physical. The eyes simply take in light, while the mind interprets the electrical impulses sent from the retina through the optic nerve to the visual cortex in the back of the brain. For this reason, much of the

Bates Method is geared toward rebuilding the connection between mind and body we all once had. Visualization exercises to help you learn to see clearer include: Ship sailing out and Runners on the track.

Analytic Vision

As Bates continually impressed upon us, an immobilized eyeball is antithetical to vision and creates watery and dim sight, and inability to see normally. Proper vision entails minimal and permanent eye movement. This analytic vision exercise is designed to help you to acquire minimum and constant eye movement.

Nutrition

Antioxidants and Vitamins are critical for optimal health. Great vision can be reached by incorporating the following:

- Vitamin A
- Vitamin E
- Vitamin C
- Antioxidants
- Omega 3 fatty acids
- Zinc
- Zeaxanthin

Foods for Better Vision

- Leafy Greens
- Eggs
- Citrus Fruits

- Seeds and Nuts
- Wild Blueberries
- Sweet Potatoes
- Fatty fish
- Non GMO Whole Grains
- Legumes
- Grass fed Beef
- Coconut Milk
- Tomatoes
- Olive Oil
- Non GMO Corn
- Pistachios
- Strawberries
- Avocados
- Peppers
- Dark Chocolate
- Coffee and Tea

Chiropractic

Living a life free of subluxation will optimize your entire body's ability to function properly including your vision. Without a good connection to the nervous system, the body can't work at optimal levels. Get your nervous system checked by a corrective chiropractor in your local area as soon as possible.

Conclusion

I hope that you found this journey through natural vision correction solutions helpful. The dietary changes along with sunning and palming were the keys to my sudden vision correction. I admit that I stopped doing the exercises once my vision improved which led to my needing to repeat the exercises two and a half years later. Isn't it nice to know that you actually can have better vision using some or all of these techniques?

If you are one that likes to dive deeper into topics of interest, I strongly recommend the books, articles and websites in the resources section.

Here's to better, clearer vision naturally!

DAILY PRACTICE

- Leave yourself notes to remind you to blink, sun, palm, swing, and to practice the other vision exercises.

- Focus weekly on one technique that you do religiously daily until it becomes second nature. Start with motion because developing a sense of motion is critical to improving your vision.
- Practice central fixation on the computer or television screen, or on what you are working on at your desk.

drjohndewitt.com

Resources

1. Lisette Scholl (2000). *28 Days to Reading without Glasses*, Citadel.
2. www.bateseyeexercises.com
3. http://integraleyesight.com/batesmethod/centralization/Fusion
4. Beilstein, Thomas J (2014-11-26). *Eyesight: How to Naturally Improve Vision - Proven Quick Tips to Improve Eyesight Vision in 30 Days or Less.*
5. http://www.chiro.org/research/ABSTRACTS/Vision_Cervical_Spine_and_Chiropractic.shtml
6. http://articles.mercola.com/sites/articles/archive/2001/07/28/coconut-health.aspx

Notes

Notes

Notes

Notes

Notes

Notes

Notes

Notes

Notes

Notes

Made in the USA
Coppell, TX
13 September 2021